マスク

behind the mask: haiku in the time of Covid-19

マスク

Edited by Margaret Dornaus

Singing Moon Press

2020

First Printing: July 2020

ISBN: 978-0-9982112-2-0

Singing Moon Press

Ozark, AR 72949

Cover Photograph: "Apple Tree & Pink Pandemic Moon"

by Djurdja Vukelic Rozic, Croatia

Footer kanji: Japanese characters for mask/masked/unmasked

マスク

Foreword

I first became acutely aware of Covid-19 in January. That's when a friend began raising concerns about a mysterious new virus taking hold in China where her daughter was serving with the Peace Corps. The threat of a dangerously amorphous epidemic—however distanced from us—was a recurring topic of concern as my friend and I charted the virus' gestation and her daughter's wellbeing in the weeks that followed.

By late February, the Peace Corps had begun considering evacuating their volunteers from China. By early March, my friend and her daughter were reunited. One crisis averted.

My friend and I, however, had no way of knowing the reach of coronavirus. By mid-March, it was clear that Covid-19 was the uninvited guest at all our tables. We watched in shock as illness and death raged throughout the world, turning much-loved centers of art and culture and humanity into locked-down ghost towns.

I began to wonder how anyone might survive this horrifying "new normal." I knew I needed someone—or something—a project of some kind, a focus—to help me endure the coming days of self-imposed isolation. I just wasn't sure who or what that might be.

Providentially, a friend from Ireland chose the moment to send me an invitation to join an online community of poets who were expressing their thoughts about the pandemic through haiku. The brainchild of Danish poet and editor Johannes S. H. Bjerg, the *Haiku in the Time of Covid-19* group was created as a safe space for haiku poets to share their responses to the novel virus on a daily basis—without criticism or judgment or any expectation beyond the recognition that the forum was a place for us to be, somehow, both together and alone. Or, as Roberta Beach Jacobson, one of the poets featured in this collection, so succinctly visualizes it

t o g e t h e r

That invitation—to experience the pandemic alone and yet together—was one of this project's early *aha* moments. More than that, it was a lifeline. When group members began tossing around the idea of creating a Covid-19 haiku anthology, my virtual hand shot up to accept another lifeline: the making of this book.

Not only do the poems presented here speak to the many challenges—loneliness, uncertainty, grief—that define the Covid-19 pandemic, they also speak to shared moments of joy and tenderness and courage. Discovering poems like this one-line haiku

life raft the answer is yes

from Anna Maris of Sweden in my inbox became a daily

pleasure, as was the arrival of Michael Nickels-Wisdom's haunting

> still
>
> six feet apart from us
>
> the coffins

sent from the United States. And offerings from India's Sanjuktaa Asopa

> today's toll
>
> higher than yesterday's . . .
>
> waxing moon

and Pravat Kumar Padhy

> lockdown—
>
> I drag my shadow away
>
> from the windowpane

Each one a lifeline.

Another lifeline appeared in the form of a haiga that Djurdja Vukelic Rozic sent me from Croatia. I instantly fell in love with the photograph: a dreamy corona moon framed by an inverted triangle of leafing branches. Would she allow me to use her beautiful picture on the anthology's cover without the accompanying haiku, I wondered. I held my breath and waited for her reply.

Rozic shared how, after weeks of lockdown, she'd caught sight of April's pink supermoon from her balcony as it traversed her family's budding apple tree. Definitely an *aha* moment. You'll find the haiku I deconstructed from her haiga on the anthology's back cover.

I knew from the beginning that I'd incorporate the name of the community that was this anthology's inspiration in the collection's title. After receiving Kathy Uyen Nguyen's lyrical haiku—the final sequence in the book—I asked if I might use her "behind the mask" line to further personalize the anthology's unique story.

Thank you to all the poets who helped make this book not simply a book of haiku but a collection of lifelines sent during this time of Covid-19. Special thanks in addition to my sister, Sara Seaman, for her support and insight as well as her invaluable proofreading skills, and for buoying my spirits along the way. I am forever grateful.

So here you are. And here I am with you. Behind the mask. Alone, *together.*

> each day a lifeline . . .
>
> and another, until *aha!*
>
> we made a book

Margaret Dornaus

July 2020

マスク

behind the mask: haiku in the time of Covid-19

マスク

Covid-19

even the full moon

shrouded in a mask

Máire Morrissey-Cummins

Ireland

counting out

five syllables

coronavirus

    Scott Wiggerman

    USA

coronavirus

makesachangefrom

anyoldvirus

    Mark Gilbert

    United Kingdom

the worm

in the apple

coronavirus

Valentina Ranaldi-Adams

USA

between me

and my worries

Coronavirus

Pere Risteski

North Macedonia

asymptomatic

a newcomer showers us

with syllables

    Hansha Teki

    New Zealand

coronavirus

trying not to think about

coronavirus

    Mark Meyer

    USA

マスク

not yet

in my spelling checker

coronavirus

Michael Dylan Welch

USA

crabgrass

coronavirus creeps

into my dreams

Claire Vogel Camargo

USA

corona deaths
crabapple blossoms touching
the windowpane

Mary White

Ireland

midnight . . .
tulips in a water glass
touching

Carol Raisfeld

USA

virus distancing—
even the daffodils
turn their heads away

John McDonald

Scotland

coronavirus
the crown
of thorns

Karen Harvey

Wales

マスク

movie after movie

the shock of people touching

each other

Myron Lysenko

Australia

Physical distance

The only thing touching

Our auras

Sandra Avrosievska

North Macedonia

マスク

flattened curves in the rise and fall of our breaths

Alegria Imperial

Canada

rising

death toll

I hold my breath

Andy McLellan

United Kingdom

マスク

starting to recover one mourning dove calls

Barbara Sabol

USA

waiting

for her lab results

the black between stars

Elliot Nicely

USA

マスク

wondering if

they'll survive the night

late frost

Elizabeth Steinglass

USA

death rates

on the rise

falling blossoms

Máire Morrissey-Cummins

Ireland

uncertain when

we will ever meet again

forget-me-nots

Olivier Schopfer

Switzerland

our visit

a window between us . . .

the warblers return

Barbara Sabol

USA

マスク

8 weeks now a crumpled origami crane

Marietta McGregor

Australia

cluster deaths

in the nursing home

forget-me-nots

Máire Morrissey-Cummins

Ireland

マスク

night shift at the morgue
a lottery ticket
in the dead man's pocket

Garry Eaton

USA

thousands gone
he doodles his heart
on a sticky note

Andrew Riutta

USA

still

six feet apart from us

the coffins

Michael Nickels-Wisdom

USA

new cluster revealed

so many saplings under

the plum tree

Myron Lysenko

Australia

daily death count . . .
wanting to believe it's all
fake news

Scott Wiggerman

USA

bent saplings
the dead pull down
the living

Steve Folkers

USA

our broken world

a lotus pod

rattles

Kath Abela Wilson

USA

life raft the answer is yes

Anna Maris

Sweden

around the world

in 80 days—

coronavirus

Susan Burch

USA

tree frogs—

I give up trying to decide

where I am

Angie Werren

USA

マスク

confined . . .
his collection of stamps
from around the world

Olivier Schopfer

Switzerland

virus washing our hands of it

Roberta Beach Jacobson

USA

マスク

as if in thanks,
the hospital's cherry blossoms
flutter through the air

Michael Dylan Welch

USA

isolation ward—
a songbird views
the cherry blossoms

Valentina Ranaldi-Adams

USA

wisps of morning
I wonder what the day
will no longer bring
    John Hawkhead
     United Kingdom

plucked daisy
all that's left
is all I am
    Terri L. French
    USA

マスク

que sera, sera . . .
my shadow's edge
begins to soften
Susan King
Wales

shut in—
the oak's eyelet shadows
on paper-thin hands
Alegria Imperial
Canada

マスク

homebound
our shadows lengthen
and merge

    Kat Lehmann

    USA

a clear view—
in the distance,
Mt. Everest

    Barbara Hay

    USA

peeking

through the curtains

everybody

Dan Burt

USA

t o g e t h e r

Roberta Beach Jacobson

USA

マスク

wildflowers
and nostalgia thrive—
while we're inside

Anne Larbes DeLorean

USA

global shutdown
the arrivals and departures
of bees in phlox

Bryan Rickert

USA

one of a crowd walking alone

Wanda Amos

Australia

isolation . . .
the white birch
sheds its skin

Mark Brager

USA

マスク

blinded by the now

we name the past

normal

Pat Davis

USA

even

at the end of the world

life goes on

Steve Folkers

USA

マスク

self-isolation

the silent birth of wind

in a sparrow

    Alegria Imperial

    Canada

        lingering day . . .

        the hush

        of inaction

           Angie Werren

           USA

isolation days
my imaginary friend
in another room

John Hawkhead
United Kingdom

too much
of a good thing—
downtime

Jean Holland
USA

マスク

all this spare time filling up a blank page

Bob Lucky

Portugal

closed book store

on display in its window

The Plague

John J. Dunphy

USA

living it while reading it dystopian fiction

Mark Meyer

USA

latest news
the growing list of books to read
before I die

Bob Lucky

Portugal

31
マスク

all morning

the zoom

of hummingbirds

    Cynthia Anderson

    USA

    sorting my thoughts

    into boxes

    midday sudoku

        Michelle Heidenrich Barnes

        USA

マスク

white butterfly
was it you who came
yesterday?
   Marietta McGregor
   Australia

   No visitors
   except for
   a neighbor's hens
      Alexis Rotella
      USA

マスク

4 p.m.—
I greet the day's first stranger
with Good Morning
        Alice Stanford
        Australia

        covid afternoon
        the cat yawns at
        my isolation
                Gregory Longenecker
                USA

light breeze—
the floral scent
of hand sanitizer

Ellen Cooper

Canada

another day of fear . . .
I donate myself
to the night breeze

Gregory Papastergiou

Greece

six feet apart—

the distance between

two caws

    Pamela Cooper

    Canada

wrapping myself

in the new normal . . .

the cold truth

    Dan Burt

    USA

マスク

all the days inside outside in my head

Marietta McGregor

Australia

time by myself

testing the possibility

of a different me

John Hawkhead

United Kingdom

マスク

two a.m.

and the cuckoo still

in isolation

Mike Gallagher

Ireland

all those watched pots

that never boil

life on the back burner

Charles Harmon

USA

マスク

morning headlines

my coffee turns

bitter

Barbara Sabol

USA

hollowing out

a coconut

the new normal

Mark Gilbert

United Kingdom

lilies of the valley—
the smell of bleach
on my hands

Angiola Inglese

Italy

online shopping
all my favourites
substituted

Marilyn Ward

United Kingdom

it seems a bit much

to Clorox

each grape

    Peggy Hale Bilbro

    USA

handy wipes

the container that won't

release them

    Peter Jastermsky

    USA

Covid drive-thru . . .
no one asks if I'd like
fries with that

Susan Burch

USA

self-isolation
a long forgotten ham
in the crisper tray

Christina Chin

Malaysia

quarantined
alone in the jar
one last olive

Pat Nelson

USA

doomsday the chocolate sold out

Alexis Rotella

USA

マスク

queuing to buy bread
the early morning sun shines
on our distancing

Gillena Cox

Trinidad

yeast so I bake

Anna Maris

Sweden

picnic for one
what do these ants know
of social distancing
    Josie Hibbing
    USA

        solo picnic
        cherry petals
        on my sandwich
            Susan Delphine Delaney
            USA

quarantine home ec

the kids learn to make

cocktails

Dan Burt

USA

stay-at-home

hokusai's great wave

in my small cup

Kath Abela Wilson

USA

quarantine treadmill I run from the numbers

Kat Lehmann

USA

quarantine birthday—
I blow out the candles
on my virtual cake

Penny Harter

USA

quarantine

the self

I can't escape from

Rachael Stanley

Ireland

quarantine . . .

a time to scatter stones

a time to gather them

Julie Warther

USA

quarantined

the brass Buddha's eyes

brighter

Jackie Chou

USA

quarantine

that homeless guy

on his regular corner

Gregory Longenecker

USA

quarantine: yr a yardbird among yard birds

Pat Nelson

USA

spring grasses—

only stray cats wander

into my yard

Angie Werren

USA

Quarantine—
a wren moves into
the empty birdhouse.
    Adele Kenny
    USA

      home quarantine
      his school backpack
      sits empty
        Judith Gorgone
        USA

another day
in quarantine
creeping buttercup

Andy McLellan
United Kingdom

home quarantine
a granddaughter's "hi"
to my "hello"

W. R. Bongcaron
Philippines

staying home
my car misses
the great outdoors

Rehn Kovacic

USA

crystal ball
the fortune-teller sees
dark clouds

Barbara Kaufmann

USA

the tiny buds
I wouldn't have noticed
shelter in place

Deborah P Kolodji

USA

shelter in place
I rearrange
the clutter

Nan Bagwell Payne

USA

more than I've ever known

about the habits of blue jays—

working from home

Agnes Eva Savich

USA

stay-at-home

a gift of rain song

from the patio

Jackie Chou

USA

マスク

sheltered in place the parakeet's mocking sound
Clifford Rames
USA

sunlight . . .
a starling takes it back
to the sky
Brendon Kent
United Kingdom

sunrise

the color of hope shelters

the sky

Marilyn Ashbaugh

USA

lockdown—

a woodpecker

knocking

Pamela Cooper

Canada

quarantined at home—

the woodpecker

goes to work

Bryan Rickert

USA

quarantine

practicing

telepathy

Luce Pelletier

Canada

corona lockdown

kitchen, living room, bedroom

and back again

    Judith Gorgone

    USA

anywhere

in the house

cat in my lap

    Agnes Eva Savich

    USA

lockdown day
making my bed
then lying in it

    Cynthia Anderson

    USA

pressing snooze
. . . again
the cat and i

    Wanda Amos

    Australia

following the sun

from one room to another . . .

lockdown

Nadejda Kostadinova

Bulgaria

isolation

in my bed making way

for a moonbeam

Josie Hibbing

USA

sudden downpour—
even in sleep I worry
about the virus

    Ram Krishna Singh

    India

the tug
of a black hole
this isolation

    Deborah P Kolodji

    USA

isolation

the scent of a distant

rose

Francesco Palladino

Italy

self-isolation

soft rain

becoming louder

Pamela A. Babusci

USA

lockdown rain if I see one more sakura haiku

Tim Gardiner

United Kingdom

isolation . . .

slowly I push

my shadow away

Praniti Gulyani

India

マスク

lockdown beard—
the colours I didn't know
I had

Dave Serjeant
United Kingdom

day three
same shirt
shaving optional

Rehn Kovacic
USA

social distancing
my hands the only thing
I've washed in days

Bob Lucky

Portugal

lockdown
setting the soft focus
for calls

Carol Judkins

USA

マスク

telemedicine day

only my top half

dressed up

Susan Delphine Delaney

USA

Zoom

a reason to get

half dressed

Jean Holland

USA

マスク

mophead hydrangeas
our Shih Tzu
needs grooming

Jackie Chou

USA

needing a trim
I FaceTime
wearing a hoodie

Jean Holland

USA

cat in heat—

whispering a love poem

over FaceTime

    Joshua Gage

    USA

    family zoom

    nobody mentions

    our bad connection

        Kat Lehmann

        USA

マスク

talk of recession—
dusk deepens
the cicadas' trill

Elliot Nicely

USA

lockdown
the cicada's pitch
a notch higher

Kinshuk Gupta

India

lockdown street
I almost hear
the evening dew

    Sanjuktaa Asopa

    India

    lockdown—
    I drag my shadow away
    from the windowpane

        Pravat Kumar Padhy

        India

lockdown every day a new bruise

Tim Gardiner

United Kingdom

lockdown silence

sighing at the pictures

of yesterday

Richa Sharma

India

first day of spring—
a new meaning
to seclusion

Michael Dylan Welch

USA

lockdown Monday
just another sparrow
in the crew

Bee Jay

Australia

leaf by leaf
my new life unfurls
pandemic spring

> Barbara Kaufmann
>
> USA

peach blossoms—
spring doesn't know
I'm at home

> Salvatore Cutrupi
>
> Italy

getting through
from one crocus
to the next

Ann K. Schwader
USA

self-isolation
pink moon in a concrete
birdbath

Sheila Windsor
United Kingdom

isolation
the moon drifts
from my view

Hemapriya Chellappan

India

decreasing
our social distance
supermoon

Ann K. Schwader

USA

today's toll
higher than yesterday's . . .
waxing moon

Sanjuktaa Asopa

India

misspent moon
sleeping away
the quarantine

Erin Castaldi

USA

crow moon
rose petals drop
onto the casket

Nancy Brady

USA

a pink moon
slips between the trees—
not touching

Sondra J. Byrnes

USA

マスク

the mask
we all wear
full moon

Olivier Schopfer

Switzerland

dark moon
even the light
stays away

David Terelinck

Australia

マスク

full moon

we take off

our masks

    Jennifer Hambrick

    USA

cloudy sky

changing masks

between stores

    Pamela A. Babusci

    USA

マスク

fashion accessory
for each pair of shoes
a matching mask

Terri L. French

USA

how things change
a sudden love
for masked strangers

Peter Jastermsky

USA

マスク

mask-to-mask—

some eyes do, some don't

smile

Alice Stanford

Australia

My mask

is better

than your mask

Alexis Rotella

USA

マスク

spring training
I practice adjusting
the strings on my mask

Margaret Dornaus

USA

spring tendrils
one string on my mask
too long

Kath Abela Wilson

USA

i doubt the words we pick could stitch   frayed strings

Alegria Imperial

Canada

coronavirus

putting the silver

back in the drawer

Tom Bierovic

USA

マスク

global pandemic:
sowing vegetable seeds,
sewing fabric masks

Barbara Hay

USA

green shoots
from unmasked stalks
spring virus

Scott Wiggerman

USA

threads and elastic
forgotten scraps recalled from
the sewing basket

Gillena Cox

Trinidad

breathing in . . .
her face a mask
of pink petals

Mark Brager

USA

pandemic
we mask
our fears

Rashmi Vesa

India

mask to mask
the eloquence
of eyes

Emanuela Nicolova

Bulgaria

87
マスク

the warmth of it . . .
her signature smile
behind a mask

Carol Judkins

USA

hiking alone—
between me and the wildlife
no masks required

Beki Reese

USA

マスク

sewing masks
startled by the thrumming
of a hummingbird

Elizabeth Steinglass

USA

family bonding
my stepson and I
make a DIY mask

Christine L. Villa

USA

no need

for a mask

the robin

  Tia Haynes

  USA

   masked fear

   the bravado in our

   video calls

    Karen Harvey

    Wales

マスク

hanging out the wash
in the warm spring sun
a row of masks

Marcyn Del Clements

USA

abandoned garden
counting the threads
of a spiderweb

Eufemia Griffo

Italy

マスク

the covid mask quarantine . . .
the dashboard spider
knits a home

Brendon Kent

United Kingdom

a quiet hour—
a spider creates
something in the corner

Nelli Slivinskaya

Germany

Pandemic—
all the old hippies
planting seeds

Pat Nelson

USA

pandemic
Mom would have been
stronger

Nan Bagwell Payne

USA

pandemic face
the slightest thing
brings tears

Barbara Hay

USA

pandemic
on the razor
dust

David Oates

USA

my neighbor's front yard
two inflatable Easter bunnies
six feet apart

John J. Dunphy

USA

hoping
for an empty tomb
pandemic Easter

Jennifer Hambrick

USA

closed church—
somewhere deep within
this need to believe

Susan King

Wales

pandemic blues
it's harder & harder
to find God

Pamela A. Babusci

USA

マスク

pandemic praying to everyone's gods

Pat Davis

USA

a crisis of faith

but, oh . . .

morning glories

Terri L. French

USA

pandemic so long as we both shall live

Margaret Dornaus

USA

pandemic . . .

blackbirds flying past

the moon

Ed Bremson

USA

haiku

in the time of Covid

the new strains

Ed Bremson

USA

covid 19

the opening

of so many hearts

Rachael Stanley

Ireland

covid war room
the slugfest of data
to flatten the curve

    Rashmi Vesa

    India

social distancing—
only our dogs
touch

    Christine L. Villa

    USA

neighborhood coyotes
I set social distancing rules
for my dog

Deborah P Kolodji

USA

social distancing
even the cat
is aloof

Dianne Moritz

USA

Still distancing—
the garden gate swings
on rusty hinges.

Adele Kenny

USA

social distancing
I stay over six feet away
from my mind

Mark Meyer

USA

social distancing—
closer than we have been
in a while

Rob Scott

Australia

my excuse
for the distance
Covid-19

Yvette Nicole Kolodji

USA

social distancing

at the tip of a branch

the beggar's cup

    Pamela Cooper

    Canada

social distancing—

again snow falls

on peonies

    Isabella Kramer

    Germany

Covid spring
eerily empty
sidewalks
Ignatius Fay
USA

the thaw . . .
our steps into summer
fragile and shaky
Djurdja Vukelic Rozic
Croatia

gone to hell

in a handbasket

summer plans

    Peggy Hale Bilbro

    USA

empty sandlot

a shadow slides

across home plate

    Elliot Nicely

    USA

マスク

silent street . . .
the occasional creak
of a wheel's shadow

Praniti Gulyani

India

a thousand starlings
inside my breath . . .
covid season

Sanjuktaa Asopa

India

CoviDazE

Sheila Windsor

United Kingdom

covid-19

. . . dandelion puffballs

awaiting a breath

John McDonald

Scotland

Covid spring . . .
a family of cats settles
beneath my car

Kanchan Chatterjee

India

a thousand ways
to wear a scarf—
Covid fashion

Luce Pelletier

Canada

マスク

Covid-19
learning to love
being alone
Lynne Jambor
Canada

coronavirus
finally realizing
i have a family
Bakhtiyar Amini
Germany

loneliness
the six feet
in between
Pat Geyer
USA

Covid-19
on the other side
the war in my dreams
Isabella Kramer
Germany

flinching

when the doorbell rings

covid-19

Tom Bierovic

USA

covid sidewalk

the optimism of children

in chalk

Gregory Longenecker

USA

covid spring—
I enter my grandchild's
Lego world

Carole MacRury

USA

a long call
to my isolated daughter . . .
hugging the phone

Myron Lysenko

Australia

heartbroken

my son's summer dreams

deferred

David Jacobson

USA

FaceTime kisses

after they hang up

I hug my iPad

Barbara Kaufmann

USA

マスク

garden visit . . .
for my deaf granddaughter,
a signed hug

Mary White

Ireland

empty swing
the echo of
children's laughter

Lynne Jambor

Canada

comics-store window

the Green Lantern sign

dark

David Oates

USA

solitude the shadow of a moth

Sheila Windsor

United Kingdom

from afar . . .
the heat and longing
of' remembered touch

Carol Raisfeld

USA

isolation
in my arms
the full moon

Francesco Palladino

Italy

together alone
forty-fifth anniversary
we are enough

Karen Harvey

Wales

fifty-fifth
wedding anniversary
we chance a kiss

Mike Gallagher

Ireland

house sparrows in love the blur of days

Claire Everett

United Kingdom

Sun patterns on the lawn—

we talk

of resilience.

Adele Kenny

USA

between solitude and loneliness the wind

social distancing
sun rays mingle
in the pine

more whisper than song bluebells

Jennifer Thompson

USA

マスク

Sequences

Another Sheltered Day

another sheltered day—
I open the window to
a robin's morning song

daily ride—
red maple buds unfurl
on either side

by the lake
a couple holding hands—
clouds cross the sun

chained playground—
crows circle above the
empty swings

food pick-up—
masked drivers line up
in the market lot

home again—
the scent of rain
before dark

       Penny Harter
       USA

Pandemica's Clouds

light rain & blackbird sing the distance of harm

breaking cloud cover counting through the strands of pandemic

the childhoodishness of antiseptic be my friend

rain clouds a leaf of i.m. books

the rebus we fish from puzzles washing hands of worship

undulatus asperatus and hole-punch cloud we remember

drifting clouds along an asphalt of ice cream summer roads of longing

Alan Summers
United Kingdom

Note: In the above sequence, "i.m." stands for "in memoriam."

Pandemic

pandemic
learning what is
essential

pandemic
angels on earth
reveal themselves

> *"Who got killed?" she cried*
> *running out of the shower*
> *to the TV set.*

pandemic
the anxiety
of extroverts

pandemic
the symptoms I feel
that I don't have

> *Early-morning Mass . . .*
> *climbing up yellow-lined steps*
> *to a bolted door.*

giving the finger
to the pandemic
magnolia spear

pandemic
the taunting yellow
of forsythia

My purchase of fish
wears yesterday's grim headlines
for undergarments

missing my parents
not missing them
pandemic

pandemic
hoarding brownies . . .
hoarding hope

pandemic
finding
glimmers

Amy Losak
Sydell Rosenberg
USA

Note: The above sequence by Amy Losak, incorporates 3 haiku by her late mother, Sydell Rosenberg, a charter member of the Haiku Society of America. In 2018, Penny Candy Books released Rosenberg's picture book *H Is For Haiku*—named a "Notable Poetry Book" by the National Council of Teachers of English in 2019.

Pandemic Fragments

morning fog, dulled mind
doors locked, windows closed, boredom
the earth will not turn

blinds open, eyes veiled
unconscious craves to be known
ghost of self reclines

green salad gone brown
empty spaces between thoughts
wood-carved white egret

chipped porcelain sink
faint hum of electric room
no after or before

red squirrel looks in
the still trees anticipate
a slight breeze bestirs

redbird raises head
molecules make rush to mate
names become numbers

Paul Austin
USA

マスク

Empty Tea Bag

covid days . . .
everything on repeat
. . . even tea

caffeine addiction—
warming up
yesterday's brew

days go by . . .
tea mold becomes
interesting

maybe it's true . . .
old tea tastes better
in a china cup

tea stains
on the tablecloth—
reading my future

Carole MacRury
USA

マスク

Covid-19 at 70

hollowed of words

       here we are then

these shapes
without form

       the whimper
       at the end of

shades
without colour

       the baby boom

*

a new dawn

       from empty caves

hunter-gatherers

       a semblance
       of similarity

in long queues

       reassembling

*

as I sleep

       unmasked
       for now

the interminable
lengthening

       our existential

of my toenails

       solitude

          Hansha Teki
          New Zealand

マスク

From Behind the Glass

morning coffee—   (BH)
caressed by a
cool breeze

dark chocolate   (MP)
a sky of blackbirds
take flight

branches   (MK)
catching branches
on the way down

pouring my heart out   (LB)
during the pandemic
the silence of deafness

self-isolation—   (CW)
a robin redbreast sings
alone

jump started   (SG)
                the crossover
today
                smell of roses
pretty much
how
it feels
                interred

sitting on damp (RC)
autumn grass
high on rotting leaves

fresh baked bread— (BH)
my sense of smell
still intact

tender bruising— (MP)
from behind the glass
an air kiss

neighbor's barbecue (MK)
smoke—
memories steeped in laughter

dappled sunlight (LB)
through the pines
speckles of hope

longing— (CW)
daffodils and tulips
poke through

backyard serenade— (RC)
fairy wrens
without aeroplanes

a kookaburra fells the dusk zoom meeting on mute (SG)

Banyan Tree Haiku Group: Barbara Hay, USA; Marianne Paul, Canada; Maggie Kennedy, USA; Leslie Bamford, Canada; Christine White, Canada; Samar Ghose, Australia; Robbie Cairns, Australia.

マスク

In the Company of Rain

in an imaginary
lighthouse

> *considerate distance?*

you complete
your diary

> *the moon*

of blank pages

> *knows*

*

wave after wave the sea will continue beyond us

Silent Week

> *days strung*

the birch
is still safe

> *on a broken*

to touch

> *guitar string*

*

132
マスク

there must be 80 ways to look out a window

silent
world?

if
only
*

midday
bells

there
you
go
*

and you find your place in the company of rain

washing up

                    evening bells

the dead
can't

                    *just
                    in time*

do
that

                    for sunset

                            Johannes S. H. Bjerg
                            Denmark

                              133
                            マスク

Another Day

wandering
from room to room—
it's only 9 a.m.

all the things
I'd planned to do—
cottonwood fluff

I put "shower"
on the calendar now—
covid-19

another day—
filing my nails down
to submission

on the list
for tomorrow—
spring rain

Sondra J. Byrnes
USA

So Many Fallen

in this sheltered park
six feet away from my dad
I hug a tree

quarantine clean
the white white paws
of my tuxedo cat

potting soil
cupped in my hands
a dream of healing herbs

chamomile tea
with just a touch of honey
my sweet antidote

midnight bird song
even the neighborhood birds
appear confused

vanilla scented pine
I sniff the bark of a tree
grateful I can smell

scarlet heart-shaped leaves
scattered on the sidewalk
so many fallen

Susan Rogers
USA

マスク

All I Need

isolation
i open the door
to the wind

river evening
social distancing
becomes me

isolation
the sounds of hours
filled with trees

self-quarantine
sometimes darkness
is all I need

Sandi Pray
USA

Behind the Mask

behind the mask
the mask I am meant
to leave behind

behind the mask
a tarot reading foretells
my loves and losses

behind the mask
my breath curls back
into myself

behind the mask
the heart that holds poetry
the lips that hold thorns

behind the mask
all the scars and stars
that unite us

Kathy Uyen Nguyen
USA

マスク

Contributors

マスク

マスク

マスク

マスク

マスク

Publication Credits

Editor's Note: *Many of the works presented in this anthology first appeared in online groups such as Haiku in the Time of Covid-19. Additional credits include the following.*

Nancy Brady, "crow moon," *Stardust Haiku 39*, March 2020.

Jackie Chou, "quarantined," The Haiku Foundation, *Haiku Dialogue,* April 8, 2020.

Claire Everett, "house sparrows . . .," *Presence 67*, July 2020.

Terri L. French, "plucked daisy," *Modern Haiku 42.3*, Autumn 2011; "a crisis of faith," *Hedgerow,* November 2018.

Praniti Gulyani, "silent street . . .," *Café Haiku* blog, May 2020.

Alegria Imperial, "i doubt the words . . ." and "flattened curves," from *we do not bleed like nightingales when felled singing,* Bones Library: Denmark, 2020.

Deborah P Kolodji, "the tiny buds," The Haiku Foundation, *Haiku Dialogue,* March 25, 2020; "the tug," *FemkuMag,* April 2020.

Amy Losak, "pandemic/the anxiety/of extroverts," *Poets and Storytellers United* (https://poetsandstorytellersunited. blogspot.com), April 17, 2020.

Anna Maris, "yeast," "life raft," *days blur*, Proletaria: Singapore, 2020.

Elliot Nicely, "waiting," *Frogpond 33.2*, "talk of recession—," *Presence 65*, "empty sandlot," *Presence 61*.

Clifford Rames, "sheltered . . .," *The Bamboo Hut 2*, 2020.

Valentina Ranaldi-Adams, "isolation ward—," Australian Haiku Society International Haiku Poetry Day, 2020.

Sydell Rosenberg, "Who got killed?," *Windchimes,* 1982; "Early morning Mass," from "Violin Case Renga," *Frogpond,* 1987; "My purchase of fish," *Modern Haiku,* 1970.

Barbara Sabol, "morning headlines," *haikuniverse,* Nov.25, 2019.

Olivier Schopfer, "uncertain when" and "confined . . .," The Haiku Foundation, *Haiku Dialogue*, April 2020; "the mask," *Stardust Haiku 22*, October 2018.

Rob Scott, "social distancing—," *Blithe Spirit 30.2.* 2020.

Hansha Teki, "hollowed of words," *Heliosparrow Poetry Journal,* May 27, 2020; "a new dawn," *Bones 20*, July 2020.

Christine L. Villa, "social distancing," Semi-finalist, New Haiku Grand Prix ITO EN, March 2020.

Kath Abela Wilson, "our broken world," *Blithe Spirit 30:2,* 2020; "stay-at-home," The Haiku Foundation, *Haiku Dialogue*, April 2020.

マスク

Margaret Dornaus

holds an MFA in the translation of poetry from the University of Arkansas. An award-winning writer, editor and teacher, her short-form poetry frequently appears in international anthologies and journals, including Red Moon Press' recently released *tanka 2020*, as well as *Contemporary Haibun Online*; *Haibun Today*; *Journeys 2015: An Anthology of International Haibun*; *MacQueen's Quinterly*; *The Red Moon Anthology of English-Language Haiku (2012-2013)*; *The Red River Book of Haibun*; and others. Examples of her free-verse poems appear in *Ain't Gonna Be Treated This Way* (Village Press); *Bearing the Mask: Southwestern Persona Poems* (Dos Gatos); *Red Earth Review; The Lindenwood Review;* and *The Texas Poetry Calendar.*

A former book review editor for the Tanka Society of America's journal *Ribbons*, Dornaus founded her small literary press, Singing Moon, in 2016 with the release of *Prayer for the Dead: Collected Haibun & Tanka Prose*—a 2017 Haiku Society of America Merit Book Award winner—and an eye toward promoting a wider audience for short-form poetry.

https://www.facebook.com/singingmoonpress

マスク

www.ingramcontent.com/pod-product-compliance
Lightning Source LLC
LaVergne TN
LVHW021341080426
835508LV00020B/2066